MW01601351

Sirtfood Diet Cookbook For Beginners

A Beginner's Sirtfood Diet Guide to Burn Fat by Activating Your "Skinny Gene" And Guarantee Your Weight Loss

Olivia Tremblay

Disclaimer Notice:

Table of Content

Introduction

Thank You For Purchasing **Sirtfood Diet Cookbook For Beginners: A Beginner's Sirtfood Diet Guide to Burn Fat by Activating Your "Skinny Gene" And Guarantee Your Weight Loss**

There is no doubt that at sirtfoods you are amazing. Nutrients and complete earth safe goods are also abundant in them.

In addition, the study has linked beneficial effects to several of the products suggested on Sirtfood Diet.

For starters, eating moderate doses of the dark chocolate with such a high amount cocoa content will decrease the danger of heart problems and help fight inflammation.

Consuming green tea will decrease the rate of stroke and diabetes and help reduce blood pressure. And turmeric has anti-inflammatory characteristics, generally having beneficial effects on the body and defending against chronic diseases related to inflammation. In humans, most Sirt foods have confirmed health benefits.

However, preliminary reports are available on the health effects of increasing amounts of a Sirtuin protein. Research in animals and cell lines has also provided interesting results. Observers have also found, for example, that high levels in worms, yeast, and mice of certain sirtuin proteins lead to longer lifespans. Sirtuin proteins alert the body during caloric restriction or fasting to burn additional fat for energy and increase insulin sensitivity. An analysis in mice showed that higher levels of Sirtuin contribute to fat loss.

Both pieces of literature suggest that sirtuins may also help suppress inflammation, prevent tumor growth, and slow the growth of Alzheimer's and high cholesterol. While experiments have shown positive results in human and mouse cell lines, the effects of increasing sirtuin levels have not been studied in human studies. Whether high levels of sirtuin protein in the body lead to longer lifespan or lower incidence of human cancer is still uncertain.

Research is currently underway to produce compounds that are successful in increasing the amounts of Sirtuin in the body. With this method, human research will begin to study the influence of sirtuins on human well-being. The results of elevated levels of a sirtuin will not be identified by then.

Breakfast Recipes

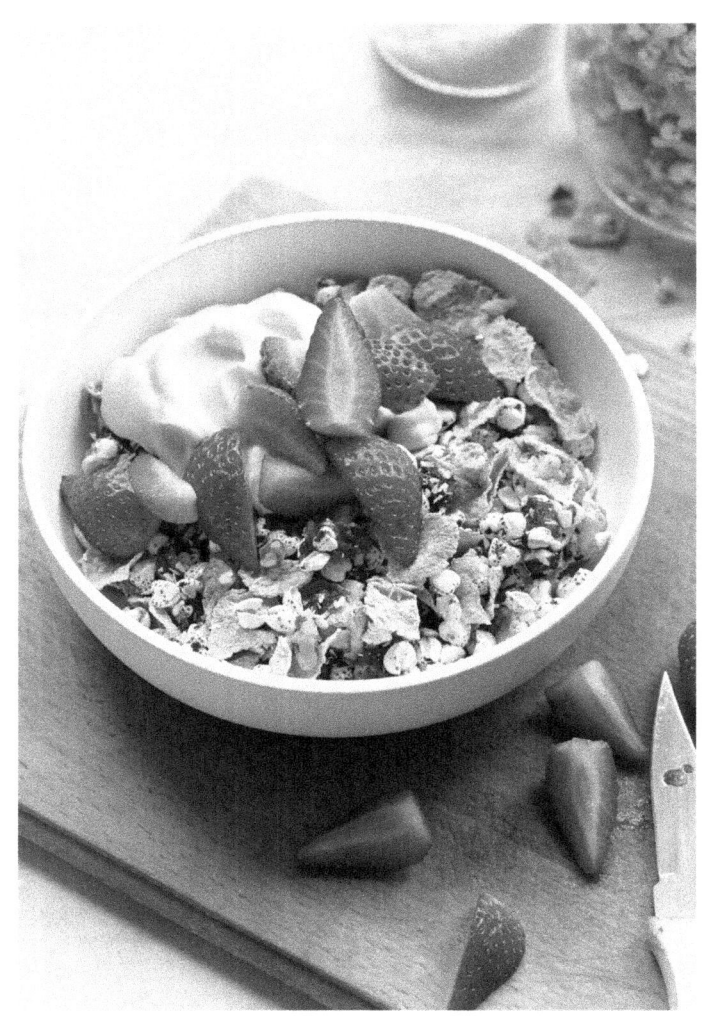

Green Omelette

(Serving: 2 Cooking time: 20 minutes, Difficulty: Normal)

234 calories

Ingredients:

- 1 shallot, peeled and finely chopped

- 2 large eggs, at room temperature

- Handful (20 g) arugula leaves

- Small handful (10 g) parsley, finely chopped

- Salt and freshly ground black pepper

Instructions:

1. Heat the oil in a large pan over medium heat and gently fry the shallot for 5 minutes.

2. Switch the heat up a bit and simmer for an extra 2 minutes. Whisk the eggs well with a fork in a bowl or cup. Before inserting the eggs, scatter the shallot equally in the skillet.

3. For either hand, turn the pan slightly so that the egg is uniformly spread.

4. Cook until the omelet sides are lifted for about a minute, and the melted egg falls into the bottom of the plate. Sprinkle

immediately and season evenly with salt and pepper over the rocket and parsley.

5. The omelet's top is still fluffy but not runny after frying, and the base is just starting to tan. Place it on a plate and taste it right now.

Savory Buckwheat Bowls

(Serving: 2, Cooking time: 30 minutes, Difficulty: Normal)

Ingredients:

- Buckwheat groats, toasted – 1 cup

- Extra virgin olive oil – 1 tablespoon

- Water – 2 cups

- Sea salt - .25 teaspoon

- Onion, diced – .5

- Button mushrooms, sliced – 4

- Parsley, chopped – 2 tablespoons

- Eggs – 2

- Capers, drained – 1 tablespoon

Instructions:

1. Rinse and transfer the buckwheat along with the water and sea salt to a saucepan. Over medium heat, cook the buckwheat groats until the water has been absorbed and the groats are fluffy. Remove from the sun, cover with a lid, and sit for 10 minutes with the groats.

2. Meanwhile, add to the pan the extra virgin olive oil and onion, along with a tiny sprinkle of sea salt. Enable the onion to cook slowly over low heat until the caramelized onion is darkened, stirring regularly. Bring in the parsley and mushrooms and saute for five minutes until the mushrooms are tender.

3. In the skillet, add the cooked buckwheat, mix it and encourage the flavors to meld and cook together for an additional two minutes.

4. When your buckwheat finishes frying, prepare your eggs in a separate pan according to your choice. Cover the cooked eggs and capers with the buckwheat, then serve immediately.

Sweet Potato and Apple Breakfast Skillet

(Serving: 4, Cooking time: 30 minutes, Difficulty: Normal)

Ingredients:

• Extra virgin olive oil – 1 tablespoon

• Apple, diced – 1 Garlic, minced – 2 cloves

• Red onion, diced – 1 Sweet potato, peeled and diced – 1

• Black pepper, ground - .25 teaspoon

• Kale, chopped – 2 cups

• Chicken apple sausage, sliced – 4 links

• Sea salt - .5 teaspoon

Instructions:

1. In a big cast iron skillet, pour the olive oil and allow it to melt over medium heat. Connect the sweet potatoes and the onion and simmer for about seven minutes, until tender.

2. In the pan, add the sliced sausage and apple, allowing it to cook for an additional five minutes, making sure to stir regularly.

3. Stir in the seasonings and kale, allowing it to cook for a few more minutes, only before the kale is wilted. Take the sweet potato skillet off the fire and serve with eggs or alone.

Cinnamon Apple Quinoa

(Serving: 2, Cooking time: 25 minutes, Difficulty: Normal)

Ingredients:

- Quinoa - .5 cup

- Water – 1.5 cups

- Apples, peeled and diced – 2

- Cinnamon – 2 teaspoons

- Sea salt - .25 teaspoon

- Honey – 2 tablespoons

Instructions:

1. To a saucepan, add the apples, quinoa, sea salt and water. Before reducing the heat to a minimum, bring the water, apples, and quinoa to a boil and cover the quinoa mixture with a lid and enable it to simmer for around twenty minutes. It is ready when the quinoa has drained the water, and the apples are tender.

2. Stir in the cinnamon and split the quinoa into two dishes for eating. Drizzle over the top of the honey before loving.

Salsa Bean Dip

Serve this zesty Salsa Bean Dip together with crackers for the next party.

(Servings: 6 Cook time: 30 minutes, Difficulty: Normal)

Ingredients:

- ½ cup. salsa
- 2 cups. canned white beans, no-salt-added, drained and rinsed
- 1 cup. low-fat cheddar, shredded
- 2 tbsps. green onions, chopped

Instructions:

1. Mix the beans with the green onions and salsa in a small pot, stir, bring to a simmer over a moderate flame, cook for 20 minutes, add cheese, stir until melted, take off heat, cool off, divide into bowls and serve.

2. Enjoy!

Chicory made from tofu and chili with arugula walnut salad

(Serving: 1 Cooking time: 30 minutes, Difficulty: Normal)

Ingredients:

- 1 teaspoon extra-virgin olive oil

- 30 g red onion, diced

- 30 g celery, diced

- 1 clove of garlic, chopped

- 1 chili, chopped

- 1 teaspoon thyme (fresh or dried)

- 1 × 400 g can of tomatoes

- 150 g silken tofu, cut into small cubes

- 1 tbsp chopped parsley

- 2 heads of chicory, quartered lengthways

For the salad:

- 35 g rocket

- 1 teaspoon capers

- 6 walnut halves, chopped

- 1 teaspoon extra-virgin olive oil

- 1 tsp balsamic vinegar

Instructions:

1. Preheat to 200 ° C / gas in the oven. 6. Heat the olive oil over medium heat in a medium-sized saucepan and cook the red onions, celery, garlic, chilies and thyme for 2-3 minutes or until tender.

2. Attach the tomatoes, and get them to a boil. With a bit of water, wash the can and dump the liquid into the bowl. For 10-15 minutes, let it boil. Attach the parsley and tofu, and be careful not to crack the tofu.

3. Put it in a baking dish with chicory. Turn it to 220 ° C / gas in the oven. 7th The seventh

4. Pour over the chicory with the hot sauce and cook for 8-10 minutes before the chicory is wilted and fried. Meanwhile, mix all the salad ingredients in a bowl and serve with the chicory.

Fried Thai Prawns

(Serving: 1 Cooking time: 10 minutes, Difficulty: Normal)

Ingredients:

- 50 g buckwheat

- 1 teaspoon ground turmeric

- 125 g chicken breast, sliced or cut into bite-sized pieces

or raw king prawns, peeled and

- deveined

- 40 g celery, cut diagonally into 1 cm slices

- 25 g of kale (weight with stems removed), cut

- 100 ml chicken broth or vegetable broth

- 4–5 basil leaves

For the stir-fry dishes:

- 30 g red onion

- 1 lemongrass stalk chopped

- 1 clove of garlic chopped1 chili, chopped1 teaspoon

ground turmeric

- 1 teaspoon ground cumin

- 1 cm fresh ginger chopped, chopped

- 1 teaspoon extra-virgin olive oil

- 1 tbsp chopped parsley

- 1 teaspoon fish sauce, soy sauce or tamari

Instructions:

1. As per the instructions on the box, cook the buckwheat, stirring the turmeric into the soup. Meanwhile, in a food processor, place all the ingredients in the paste and flash before you have a smooth paste. If you don't have a food processor, just cut it all as thinly and blend well as you can.

2. Over low melt, heat the paste in a pan. The celery and kale, add the chicken or shrimp and cook for 4 to 5 minutes or until the chicken or shrimp are finished.

3. Connect the broth, then simmer for 1-2 more minutes. Halve the leaves from the basil and apply them to the pan.

4. Serve with the buckwheat.

Black currants and oat yogurt

(Serving: 2 Cooking time: 15 minutes, Difficulty: Easy)

Ingredients:

- 100 g black currants, washed and stems removed

- 2 tbsp powdered sugar + 100 ml water

- 200 g natural yogurt

- 40 g jumbo oats

Instructions:

1. In a small skillet, add the black currants, sugar and water and bring to a boil. Slightly reduce the heat, boil vigorously and continue to cook for 5 minutes.

2. Turn the stove off and allow it to cool down. It is now easy to refrigerate the blackcurrant compote before it is used. Place the yogurt in a wide bowl with the oats and whisk together.

3. Divide between two bowls of blackcurrant compote and cover with yogurt and oats. To toss the compote through the yogurt, use a cocktail stick.

Mung Sprouts Salsa

A good, savory salsa with sprouts and corn

(Servings: 2 Cook time: 10 minutes, Difficulty: Normal)

Ingredients:

- 1 red onion, chopped 2 c. mung beans, sprouted

- A pinch of red chili powder

- 1 green chili pepper, chopped

- 1 tomato, chopped

- 1 tsp. chat masala

- 1 tsp. lemon juice

- 1 tbsp. coriander, chopped Black pepper to the taste

Instructions:

1. Mix the onion with the mung sprouts, chili pepper, cabbage, chili pepper, and chili pepper in a salad dish. Chaat masala powder, lemon juice, cilantro and pepper, toss together, break into small cups.

Main Dishes Recipes

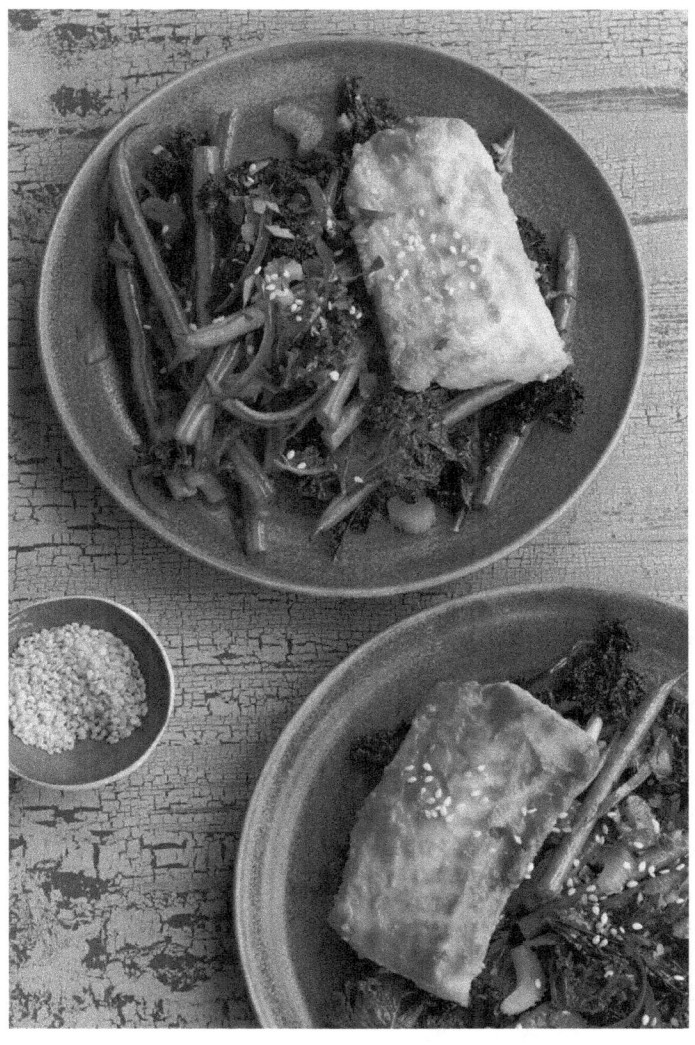

Salmon buckwheat Pasta

(Serving: 4 Cook Time: 25 Minutes, Difficulty: Normal)

Ingredients:

- 300 g skinless salmon fillet

- 1 teaspoon extra-virgin olive oil

- 250 g buckwheat noodles

- 100 g kale, chopped

- 1 large zucchini, quarter lengthways

- Cut 1 red onion into slices

- Cut 4 cloves of garlic into slices

- 1 tbsp Herbs of Provence

- 1 tbsp extra-virgin olive oil

For the sauce:

- 650 ml milk or dairy-free alternative

- 65 g unsalted butter   - 65 g buckwheat or flour

- 150 g cheddar cheese, grated

- 2 tbsp chopped parsley   2 tbsp capers

Instructions:

1. Heat 200 C / gas in the oven. 6. Rub the salmon with olive oil and put it on a sheet of foil. To get a box, fold over the sides and seal them. Bake for 15 minutes in the oven. Cook the pasta on the box according to the instructions.

2. Keep it from sticking, rinse, then spill some warm water out of the kettle and set it aside. Bring the milk to a boil in a shallow saucepan to make the sauce, being careful not to overflow it. Then in a separate pan, heat the butter and add the flour. Until you have a combination, mix them.

3. Cook gently for 30 seconds to 1 minute on low heat. Add the hot milk steadily, continually stirring, until you've got a good thick sauce. Remove from the heat and apply 100 g of cheese, parsley and capers. Meanwhile, sear the kale or steam it until tender. Cook the zucchini, red onion, garlic and herbs in olive oil in a skillet over medium heat for 2-3 minutes, until tender. Mix with the kale that has been roasted.

4. At the maximum temperature, heat a barbecue. Peel the cooked salmon and blend, put in an ovenproof bowl and scatter over the remaining cheese with the pasta, cooked vegetables and sauce.

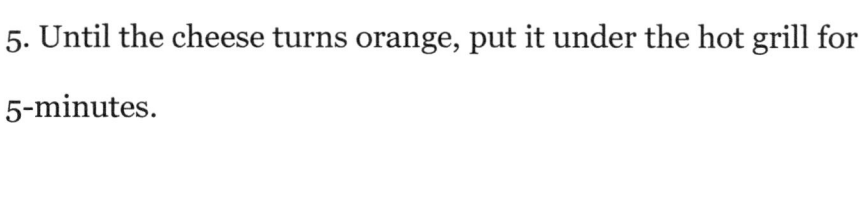

5. Until the cheese turns orange, put it under the hot grill for 5-minutes.

Brown Basmati Rice Pilaf

(Servings: 2 Cook time: 13 minutes, Difficulty: Normal)

Ingredients:

- ½ tbsp. vegan butter

- ½ c. mushrooms, chopped

- ½ c. brown basmati rice

- 3 tbsps. water

- 1/8 tsp. dried thyme

- Ground pepper to taste

- ½ tbsp. olive oil

- ¼ c. green onion, chopped 1 c. vegetable broth

- ¼ tsp. salt ¼ c. chopped, toasted pecans

Instructions:

1. Over medium-low pressure, position a saucepan. Add the oil and butter.

2. When it melts, mushrooms are added and cook until tender.

3. Stir in the brown rice and the green onion. For 3 minutes, cook. Revolve endlessly.

4. Incorporate the soup, sugar, salt and thyme.

5. Lower the heat and cover it with a cap as it starts to bubble. Simmer until it is prepared with rice. If ordered, add more water or broth.

6. Add the pecans and vinegar, stirring.

7. Serve.

Char-grilled beef with a red wine jus, onion rings, garlic kale, and herb-roasted potatoes

(Serving: 1, Cooking time: 30 Minutes, Difficulty: Normal)

Ingredients:

• 1 / 2 cup (100g) potatoes, peeled and cut into 3 / 4 -inch (2cm) diced pieces

• 1 tablespoon extra-virgin olive oil

• 2 tablespoons (5g) parsley, finely chopped

• 1 / 3 cup (50g) red onion, sliced into rings

• 2 ounces (50g) kale, sliced

• 2 garlic cloves, finely chopped

• 1 x 4- to 5-ounce (120 to 150g) beef tenderloin (about 1 1 / 2 inch or 3.5cm thick) or sirloin steak (3 / 4 inch or 2cm thick)

• 3 tablespoons (40ml) red wine

• 5 / 8 cup (150ml) beef stock

• 1 teaspoon tomato purée

• 1 teaspoon corn flour, dissolved in

• 1 tablespoon water

Instructions:

1. Heat the oven to 220oC (425oF). Place the potatoes in a boiling water saucepan, bring to a boil again and simmer for 4 to 5 minutes, then drain. Put 1-teaspoon of oil in the roasting pan and roast for 35 to 45 minutes in the hot oven. Switch the potatoes and make sure they cook evenly after 10 minutes.

2. Remove from the oven until baked, sprinkle with chopped parsley, and blend properly. Over medium heat, fry the onion in 1 teaspoon of oil for 5 to 7 minutes, until soft and nicely caramelized. Just stay wet. For 2 to 3 minutes, steam the kale, then rinse. Gently fry the garlic in 1/2 teaspoon of oil, until soft but not browned, for 1 minute. Attach the kale and fry for an extra 1 to 2 minutes, until tender. Just stay wet.

3. Over high pressure, heat an ovenproof frying pan before you smoke. Coat the meat in 1/2 teaspoon of the oil and fry it over medium-high heat in the hot pan as you want the meat done (see our cooking time guide). It would be easier to sear it and then move the pan to an oven set at 425oF (220oC) if you prefer the meat medium and finish the cooking that way for the specified times.

4. Set aside to rest and remove the meat from the pan. To put in some meat residue, add the wine to the hot pan. Simmer to decrease the wine by half until the wine is syrupy and tastes concentrated. In the steak pan, add the stock and tomato purée and bring to a boil, then add the paste of corn-flour to thicken the sauce, adding it a little at a time until you get the consistency you like.

5. Stir in any of the juices from the rested steak, and serve with the roasted potatoes, kale, onion rings, and red wine sauce.

Kidney bean mole with baked potato

(Serving: 1, Cooking time: 25 Minutes, Difficulty: Normal)

Ingredients:

- 1 / 4 cup (40g) red onion, finely chopped

- 1 teaspoon finely chopped fresh ginger

- 2 garlic cloves, finely chopped

- 1 Thai chili, finely chopped

- 1 teaspoon extra-virgin olive oil

- 1 teaspoon ground turmeric

- 1 teaspoon ground cumin pinch of ground clove pinch

of ground cinnamon

- 1 medium baking potato

- 7 / 8 cup (190g) canned chopped tomatoes

- 1 teaspoon brown sugar

- 1 / 3 cup (50g) red bell pepper, cored, seeds removed,

and roughly chopped

- 5 / 8 cup (150ml) vegetable stock

- 1 tablespoon cocoa powder

- 1 teaspoon sesame seeds

- 2 teaspoons peanut butter (smooth if available, but chunky is fine)

- 7 / 8 cup (150) canned kidney beans

- 2 tablespoons (5g) parsley, chopped

Instructions:

1. Heat the oven to 200oC (400°F). In a medium saucepan over medium heat, fry the onion, ginger, garlic, and chili in the oil for about 10 minutes until tender. Attach the seasoning, then simmer for 1 to 2 more minutes.

2. Place the potato in the hot oven on a baking tray and bake for 45 to 60 minutes, until the middle is soft (or longer, depending on how crispy the outside maybe).

3. Meanwhile, add to the saucepan the tomatoes, cinnamon, red pepper, stock, cocoa powder, sesame seeds, peanut butter, and kidney beans and gently simmer for 45 to 60 minutes. To end, sprinkle with the parsley.

5. Break the potato in half and serve on top with the mole.

Cauliflower Kale curry

(Serving: 4 Cook Time: 30 Minutes, Difficulty: Normal)

Ingredients:

- 200 g buckwheat
- 2 tbsp ground turmeric
- 1 red onion, chopped
- 3 cloves of garlic, minced
- 2.5 cm piece of fresh ginger, chopped
- 1–2 chili peppers, chopped
- 1 tbsp coconut oil 1 tbsp mild curry powder
- 1 tbsp ground cumin
- 2 × 400 g cans of chopped tomatoes
- 300 ml vegetable broth
- 200 g kale, roughly chopped
- 300 g cauliflower, chopped
- 1 × 400 g can of butter beans, drained
- 2 tomatoes, cut into wedges
- 2 tbsp chopped coriander

Instructions:

1. As per the instructions on the box, cook the buckwheat and apply 1-tablespoon of turmeric to the bath. Meanwhile, fry the onion, garlic, ginger, and chili peppers over medium heat for 2-3 minutes in the coconut oil.

2. Apply the seasonings, like the remaining tablespoon of turmeric, and continue to cook for 1–2 minutes over low to medium heat.

3. Add the canned tomatoes and broth and bring to a boil for 10 minutes, then simmer.

4. Cook for 10 minutes and add the broccoli, cauliflower and butter beans.

5. Attach the coriander and the tomato wedges and simmer for another minute. Then feed the buckwheat with them.

Kidney bean burritos

(Serving: 4 Cook Time: 45 minutes, Difficulty: Normal)

Ingredients:

- 1 tbsp extra-virgin olive oil

- 1 red onion, diced

- 3 cloves of garlic, chopped

- 1 tablespoon chili, chopped

- 1 tbsp paprika

- 1 tbsp ground cumin

- 1 teaspoon chili powder

- 1 tbsp chopped coriander

- 2 tomatoes, chopped

- 3 × 400 g cans of kidney beans, drained

- 500 ml vegetable broth

- 150 g cheddar or vegan cheese

- 8 whole grain tortilla wraps

- 1 × 500 g glass of tomato passata

- 1 × 200 g jar of jalepeño peppers (optional)

For the salad:

- 125 g rocket   1 paprika,

- 3 tomatoes sliced ½ small red onion sliced

- 1 avocado cut into slices, peeled and sliced

- 1 tablespoon of extra-virgin olive oil

- juice ½ lemon

Instructions:

1. Over medium heat, heat a large saucepan. Apply the olive oil and sauté for 1-2 minutes with the onion, garlic and chili, until slightly softer. Add the coriander and spices and simmer for another 1–2 minutes. Tomatoes, kidney beans and broth are added. Bring it to a boil and simmer for 20 minutes over medium-high heat. You want it to evaporate more of the oil. So, keep an eye out for them and stir regularly.

2. Take the stove off and allow it to cool off a little. Take about a third of the pan with the kidney beans and set aside. Soften the remaining mixture in a food processor or mixer, then return to the plate, add the whole beans and whisk in. It should be a little rigid in the mixture. Allowing it to cool fully would make wrapping the burritos smoother.

3. Heat 200 C / gas in the oven. 6th On top of the wraps, spread the cheese; keep back a bit to spread over the top at the end. Divide the filling and roll each into a sausage tin between the wraps. On the bottom of an ovenproof bowl wide enough to accommodate all the burritos in a single layer, spread a thin layer of passata.

4. Place them in this direction and drizzle over them with the remaining passata. If used, sprinkle the remaining cheese and the jalapeños with it.

5. Cover the bowl with foil, then bake for 20-25 minutes in the oven. To brown the cheese, cut the foil and bake for another 5 minutes. Throw in all the salad ingredients and serve with the heated burritos.

Miso and Sesame Glazed Tofu with Ginger and Chili Stir-Fried Greens

(Serving: 1, Cooking time: 25 Minutes, Difficulty: Normal)

Ingredients:

*   1 tablespoon mirin

*   3 1 / 2 teaspoons (20g) miso paste

*   1 x 5-ounce (150g) block of firm tofu

*   1 stalk (40g) celery, trimmed (about 1 / 3 cup when sliced)

*   1 / 4 cup (40g) red onion, sliced

*   1 small (120g) zucchini (about 1 cup when sliced)

*   1 Thai chili 2 garlic cloves

*   1 teaspoon finely chopped fresh ginger

*   3 / 4 cup (50g) kale, chopped

*   2 teaspoons sesame seeds

*   1 / 4 cup (35g) buckwheat

*   1 teaspoon ground turmeric

*   2 teaspoons extra-virgin olive oil

*   1 teaspoon tamari (or soy sauce, if you are not avoiding gluten)

Instructions:

1. Heat the oven to 200oC (400oF). Using parchment paper to cover a small roasting pan. Mix mirin and miso.

2. Break the tofu lengthwise, then diagonally cut each slice in half into triangles. With the miso paste, coat the tofu and leave to marinate while cooking the other ingredients. At an angle, dice the celery, red onion, and zucchini.

3. Slice the chili, garlic and ginger thinly and set aside. In a steamer, cook the kale for 5 minutes. Withdraw and put aside. In the roasting pan, put the tofu, scatter the sesame seeds over the tofu, and roast for 15 to 20 minutes in the oven, until the tofu is nicely caramelized. Wash the buckwheat in a sieve, then put it along with the turmeric in a pan of boiling water.

4. Cook according to the instructions in the box, then rinse. Heat the oil in a frying pan; add the celery, onion, zucchini, chili, garlic and ginger when heated, and fry for 1 to 2 minutes on high heat, then reduce to medium heat for 3 to 4 minutes until the vegetables are cooked through but still crunchy. If the vegetables stick to the plate, you will need to apply a tablespoon of water. Connect the tamari and kale and simmer for an additional minute. Serve with the greens and buckwheat when the tofu is ready.

Sirt super salad

(Serving: 1, Cooking time: 25 Minutes, Difficulty: Normal)

Ingredients:

- 1 3 / 4-ounce (50g) arugula

- 1 3 / 4-ounce (50g) endive leaves

- 3 1 / 2 ounces (100g) smoked salmon slices

- 1 / 2 cup (80g) avocado, peeled, stoned, and sliced

- 1 / 2 cup (50g) celery including leaves, sliced

- 1 / 8 cup (20g) red onion, sliced

- 1 / 8 cups (15g) walnuts, chopped

- 1 tablespoon capers

- 1 large Medjool date, pitted and chopped

- 1 tablespoon extra-virgin olive oil

- juice of 1 / 4 lemon

- 1 / 4 cup (10g) parsley, chopped

Instructions:

1. Place the salad leaves on a plate or in a large bowl.

2. Mix all the remaining ingredients together and serve on top of the leaves.

Variations:

- Replace the smoked salmon with 1 1 / 3 cup (100g) canned green lentils or cooked Le Puy lentils for a lentil Sirt super salad.

- Replace the smoked salmon with a sliced fried chicken breast for a chicken Sirt super salad.

- According to preference, simply substitute the smoked salmon with canned tuna (in water or oil) for a tuna Sirt super salad.

Turkey escalope with sage, capers, and parsley and spiced cauliflower "couscous"

(Serving: Cooking time: 20 Minutes, Difficulty: Normal)

Ingredients:

• 1 1 / 2-cups (150g) cauliflower, roughly chopped

• 2 garlic cloves, finely chopped

• 1 / 4 cup (40g) red onion, finely chopped

• 1 Thai chili, finely chopped 1 teaspoon finely chopped

fresh ginger 2 tablespoons extra-virgin olive oil

• 2 teaspoons ground turmeric

• 1 / 2 cup (30g) sun-dried tomatoes, finely chopped

• 1 / 4 cup (10g) fresh parsley, chopped

• 1 / 3-pound (150g) turkey cutlet or steak (see above)

• 1 teaspoon dried sage

• juice of 1 / 4 lemon 1 tablespoon capers

Instructions:

1. Place the raw cauliflower in a food processor to create the "couscous." Pulse to finely slice the cauliflower in 2-second bursts until it resembles couscous.

2. Alternatively, you should only use a knife to finely cut it. Fry the garlic, red onion, chili, and ginger until tender but not browned in 1 teaspoon of the oil. Connect the cauliflower and turmeric and simmer for 1 minute.

3. Remove and add the sun-dried tomatoes and half of the parsley from the heat. Use the remaining oil in a frying pan over medium heat for 5 to 6 minutes, rotate periodically, and then coat the turkey escalope in the salvia and a little oil.

4. Apply the lemon juice, remaining parsley, capers, and 1-tablespoon of water to the pan when cooked. It would make a sauce for the cauliflower to serve.

Courgette Risotto

(Servings: 8 Cook time: 18 minutes, Difficulty: Normal)

Ingredients:

- 2 tbsps. olive oil 4 cloves garlic, finely chopped

- 1.5 lb. Rice (Arborio) 6 tomatoes, chopped

- 2 tsps. chop rosemary

- 6 courgettes, finely diced

- 1 ¼ c. peas, fresh or frozen

- 12 c. hot vegetable stock 1 c. chopped

- Salt and ground black pepper to taste

Instructions:

1. Over medium heat, position a big heavy-bottomed pan. Apply the oil.

2. Add the onion and sauté until transparent when the oil is heated.

3. Cook the tomatoes until they're tender. Stir in the rice and the rosemary next. Mix thoroughly. Half the stock is added and cooked until dry. Stir occasionally.

4. Add the remaining stock and cook for about 3-4 minutes.

5. Attach the zucchini and peas and simmer until the rice is tender.

6. To taste, add salt and pepper.

7. Stir in the basil, then quit for 5 minutes to sit down.

8. Serve warm and enjoy

Thai Red Curry

(Servings: 4 Cook time: 1 hour and 15 minutes, Difficulty: Normal)

Ingredients:

- 1 ½ c. packed thinly sliced kale
- Pinch of salt, more to taste
- 2 tbsps.
- Thai red curry paste
- 1 tbsp. soy sauce
- 1 ¼ c. long-grain brown jasmine rice
- 1 small white onion, chopped
- 1 tbsp. grated ginger
- 1 red bell pepper
- 1 tbsp. coconut oil or olive oil
- ½ c. water
- 1 ½ tsps. coconut sugar or turbinado sugar
- 2 cloves garlic
- 2 tsps. lime juice
- 3 carrots, peeled and sliced
- 1 bell pepper 1 can (14 oz.) regular coconut milk

Instructions:

1. Bring a big pot of water and bring it to a boil to make rice. To avoid excess, insert the rinsed rice and begin to boil for 30 minutes, reducing heat when necessary. Drain the rice, remove it from the sun, and place the rice back in the tank. Cover and let the rice sit for 10 minutes or longer until you are ready to eat. Just before eating, season the rice with salt and fluff it with a fork to taste.

2. Fire up a large skillet over the medium fire with the deep sides to make the curry, then add your oil until warm. Then add the onion and a sprinkle of salt and simmer until the onion has softened and becomes translucent, continually stirring for about 5 minutes. Garlic and ginger are introduced and cook for around 25-30 seconds while continually stirring until fragrant.

3. Attach the carrots and your bell peppers, roast, occasionally stirring, 3 to 5 minutes more, until these bell peppers are fork-tender. Then add your curry paste and simmer, constantly stirring, for around 2 minutes.

4. To blend, add water, kale, coconut milk and sugar and whisk. Bring the mixture to a boil over a medium flame. To maintain a moderate simmer, reduce the flame as required and cook until the carrots, peppers, and kale have softened to your taste, stirring for around 5-10 minutes periodically.

5. Take the pot from the blaze and season with tamari and rice vinegar. To taste, add salt (for the best flavor). If a little more energy is needed for your curry, add 1/2 teaspoon more tamari, or add 1/2 teaspoon more rice vinegar for more acidity. Divide the curry and rice into bowls and garnish with sliced cilantro and a splash of red pepper flakes, if you prefer. Serve on the side if you prefer hot curries, with sriracha or chili garlic sauce.

6. If you want to add tofu, first bake it and add coconut milk to it. It would eat up too much of the fat if you add raw tofu, so baking it will considerably increase the taste, anyway.

Side Dish Recipes

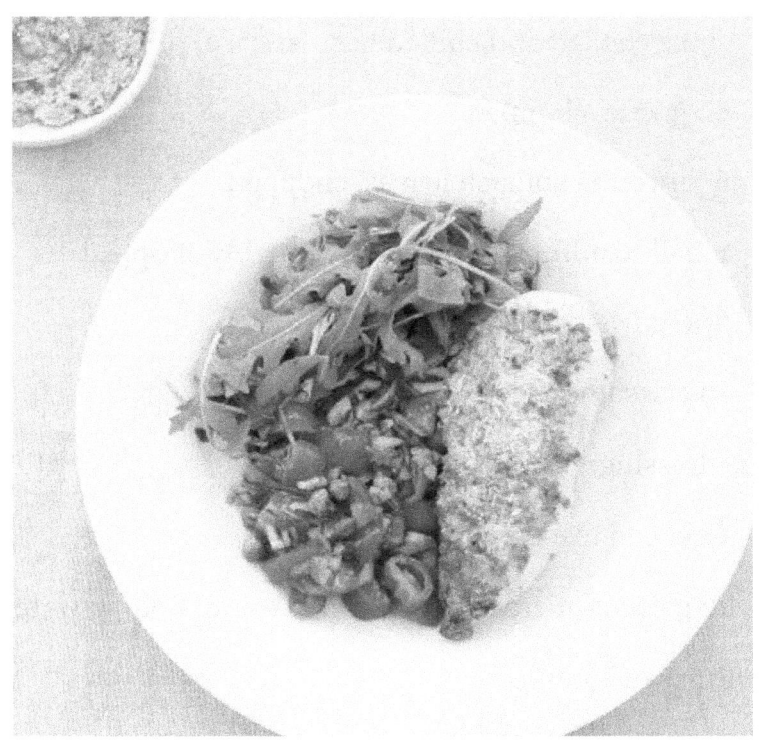

Roast Chicken Kale Salad with peanut dressing

(Serving: 2, Cooking time: 20 Minutes, Difficulty: Normal)

Ingredients:

- 60 g small broccoli florets

- 150 g cooked and chilled basmati rice

- 60 g kale, chopped

- 60 g young spinach leaves, chopped

- Small handful (10 g) parsley, roughly chopped

- 200 g fried chicken breast, cut

- 10 g sesame seeds

For the dressing:

- 1 heaped teaspoon peanut butter

- 10 g coconut cream dissolved in 30 ml boiling water

- Juice of ½ lime

- ½ teaspoon brown sugar

- ½ teaspoon sesame oil

Instructions:

1. Steam the broccoli over a pan of boiling water for 5 minutes or until just tender.

2. Put the rice in a large bowl and use a fork to break up any lumps. Add the kale, spinach, broccoli and parsley and stir gently. Add the dissolved coconut to the peanut butter one at a time. Stir each time to ensure an even consistency.

3. Add the lime juice, brown sugar, and sesame oil. Divide the dressing in half and pour one half over the rice and vegetables and stir. Pour the rest of the dressing over the cooked chicken and stir gently until the chicken is completely coated. Scoop the dressed chicken over the vegetables and serve with the sesame seeds sprinkled on top.

Rosemary Endives

(Servings: 2 Cook time: 30 minutes, Difficulty: Easy)

Ingredients:

- 2 tbsps. Olive oil

- 1 tsp. dried rosemary

- 2 halved endives

- ¼ tsp. black pepper

- ½ tsp. turmeric powder

Instructions:

1. In a baking pan, combine the endives with the oil and the other ingredients, toss gently, introduce in the oven and bake at 400 0F for 20 minutes. Divide between plates and serve.

Scallops with Almonds and Mushrooms

(Servings: 4 Cook time: 15 Minutes, Difficulty: Easy)

Ingredients:

- 1 lb. scallops

- 2 tbsps. olive oil

- 4 scallions, chopped

- ½ c. mushrooms, sliced

- 2 tbsps. almonds, chopped

- 1 c. coconut cream

Instructions:

1. Heat up a pan with the oil over medium heat; add the scallions and the mushrooms and sauté for 2 minutes.

2. Add the scallops cook over medium heat for 8 minutes more, divide into bowls and serve.

Buckwheat Noodles with Chicken Kale & Miso Dressing

(Serving: 2, Cooking time: 30 Minutes, Difficulty: Normal)

Ingredients:

For the noodles:

• 2-3 handfuls of kale leaves (removed from the stem and roughly cut)150 g / 5 oz buckwheat noodles (100% buckwheat, no wheat)

• 3-4 shiitake mushrooms, sliced

• 1 teaspoon coconut oil or ghee

• 1 brown onion, finely diced

• 1 medium free-range chicken breast, sliced or diced

• 1 long red chilli, thinly sliced (seeds in or out depending on how hot you like it)

• 2 large garlic cloves, finely diced

• 2-3 tablespoons Tamari sauce (gluten-free soy sauce)

For the miso dressing:

• 1½ tablespoon fresh organic miso

• 1 tablespoon Tamari sauce

• 1 tablespoon extra-virgin olive oil

- 1 tablespoon lemon or lime juice

- 1 teaspoon sesame oil (optional)

Instructions:

1. Bring a medium saucepan of water to boil. Add the kale and cook for 1 minute, until slightly wilted. Remove and set aside but reserve the water and bring it back to the boil. Add the soba noodles and cook according to the package instructions (usually about 5 minutes). Rinse under cold water and set aside.

2. In the meantime, pan fry the shiitake mushrooms in a little ghee or coconut oil (about a teaspoon) for 2-3 minutes, until lightly browned on each side. Sprinkle with sea salt and set aside.

3. In the same frying pan, heat more coconut oil or ghee over medium-high heat. Sauté onion and chilli for 2-3 minutes and then add the chicken pieces. Cook 5 minutes over medium heat, stirring a couple of times, then add the garlic, tamari sauce and a little splash of water. Cook for a further 2-3 minutes, stirring frequently until chicken is cooked through.

4. Finally, add the kale and soba noodles and toss through the chicken to warm up.

5. Mix the miso dressing and drizzle over the noodles right at the end of cooking, this way you will keep all those beneficial probiotics in the miso alive and active.

Asian King Prawn Stir-Fry with Buckwheat

(Serving: 4, Cooking time: 40 Minutes, Difficulty: Normal)

Ingredients:

- 150g shelled raw king prawns, deveined

- 2 tsp tamari (you can use soy sauce if you are not

avoiding gluten)

- 2 tsp extra-virgin olive oil

- 75g soba (buckwheat noodles)

- 1 garlic clove, finely chopped

- 1 bird's eye chilli, finely chopped

- 1 tsp finely chopped fresh ginger

- 20g red onions, sliced

- 40g celery, trimmed and sliced

- 75g green beans, chopped 50g kale, roughly chopped

- 100ml chicken stock 5g lovage or celery leaves

Instructions:

Heat a frying pan over a high heat, then cook the prawns in 1 teaspoon of the tamari and 1 teaspoon of the oil for 2–3 minutes. Transfer the prawns to a plate. Wipe the pan out with kitchen paper, as you're going to use it again.

Cook the noodles in boiling water for 5–8 minutes or as directed on the packet. Drain and set aside.

Meanwhile, fry the garlic, chilli and ginger, red onion, celery, beans and kale in the remaining oil over a medium–high heat for 2–3 minutes. Add the stock and bring to the boil, then simmer for a minute or two, until the vegetables are cooked but still crunchy.

Add the prawns, noodles and lovage/celery leaves to the pan, bring back to the boil then remove from the heat and serve.

Smoked trout salad

(Serving: 2, Cooking time: 20 Minutes, Difficulty: Normal)

Ingredients:

- 200 g new potatoes, halved

- 50 g rocket

- 50 g young spinach leaves

- 50 g watercress

- 8 radishes, cut and quartered

- Large handful (20 g) parsley, roughly chopped

- 100 g red seedless grapes, halved

- 130 g smoked trout, thinly sliced

For the dressing:

- 1 tbsp mayonnaise

- 1 tbsp natural yogurt

- 1 teaspoon olive oil

- 2 teaspoons capers, chopped

- 2 cocktail cucumbers, finely chopped

Instructions:

1. Steam the new potatoes for 15 to 20 minutes until tender.

2. In a large bowl, mix the rocket, spinach, watercress, new potatoes, radishes and parsley. Mix mayonnaise, yogurt, olive oil, capers, pickles and lemon juice to make a dressing. Stir half of the dressing into the greens.

3. Arrange the lettuce and potato on two serving plates. Distribute the grapes and smoked trout evenly on the plates.

Quick & Easy Recipes

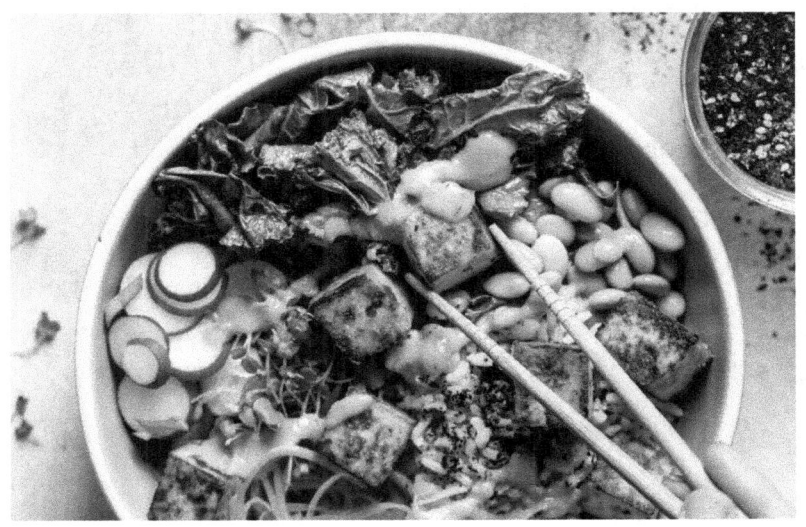

Chocolate cupcakes with matcha Icing

(Serving: 10-12, Cooking time: 35 Minutes, Difficulty: Normal)

Ingredients:

- 150g self-raising flour

- 200g caster sugar

- 60g cocoa

- ½ tsp salt

- ½ tsp fine coffee espresso, decaf whenever liked

- 120ml milk

- ½ tsp vanilla concentrate

- 50ml vegetable oil

- 1 egg

- 120ml bubbling water

For the icing:

- 50g margarine, at room temperature

- 50g icing sugar

- 1 tbsp matcha green tea powder

- ½ tsp vanilla bean paste

- 50g delicate cream cheese

Instructions:

1. Preheat the oven to 180C/160C fan. Line a cupcake tin with paper or silicone cake cases.

2. Place the flour, sugar, cocoa, salt, and coffee powder in an enormous bowl and blend completely.

3. Add the milk, vanilla concentrate, vegetable oil, and egg to the dry ingredients and utilize an electric blender to beat until very much joined. Cautiously pour in the bubbling water gradually and beat on a low speed until completely combined. Utilize a high speed to beat for a further moment to add air to the batter. The batter is significantly more liquid than a typical cake blend. Have confidence, it will taste astonishing!

4. Spoon the batter uniformly between the cake cases. Each cake case ought to be close to ¾ full. Heat in the oven for 15-18 minutes, until the blend bobs back when tapped. Remove from the oven and permit to cool totally before icing.

5. To make the icing, cream the margarine and icing sugar together until it's pale and smooth. Include the matcha powder and vanilla and mix once more. At long last include the cream cheese and beat until smooth. Channel or spread over the cakes.

SIRT Food Mushroom Scramble Eggs

(Serving: 4, Cooking time: 30 Minutes, Difficulty: Normal)

Ingredients:

- 2 eggs 1 tsp ground turmeric

- 1 tsp gentle curry powder

- 20g kale, generally hacked

- 1 tsp additional virgin olive oil

- ½ 10,000-foot stew, daintily cut

- handful of catch mushrooms, daintily cut

- 5g parsley, finely hacked

- *optional* Add a seed blend as a topper and some

Rooster Sauce for flavor

Instructions:

1. Mix the turmeric and curry powder and include a little water until you have accomplished a light paste.

2. Steam the kale for 2–3 minutes.

3. Heat the oil in a pan over a medium warmth and fry the stew and mushrooms for 2–3 minutes until they have begun to brown and mellow.

Tandoori spears

(Serving: 2, Cooking time: 15 Minutes, Difficulty: Normal)

Ingredients:

• 4 wooden skewers Soaked in water for 30 minutes

• 400 g firm tofu, cut into large cubes

• 3 tsp tandoori masala powder (dry tandoori spice mixture)

• 1 teaspoon of ground turmeric

• juice from 1 lime Salt and freshly ground black pepper

• 1 red onion, cut into large slices

• 1 pepper, deseeded and cut into large pieces

• 100 g natural yogurt

• Large amount (20 g) parsley, roughly chopped

Instructions:

1. Spread the tofu on a plate with kitchen paper. Cover with kitchen paper and set aside.

2. Mix the tandoori masala, turmeric, lime juice and lots of salt and pepper together.

3. Add the tofu pieces, stir until completely coated and let sit for 5 minutes.

4. Heat the grill on high. Cover the grill tray with a piece of foil (turned up at the edges to catch juices). Prepare four equal skewers by threading a piece of onion, tofu, and bell pepper. You should get two sets of onion, tofu, and bell pepper on each skewer.

5. Make sure the ingredients aren't squeezed too much. The rest of the marinade with yogurt and fresh parsley Mix Gently brush this onto all of the skewers on all sides.

6. Place on the prepared grill tray. Place under the hot grill for about 5 minutes until one side is brown, then turn and cook for another 5 minutes, until everything is cooked through and the vegetables are soft and slightly charred.

Stuffed avocado with chicken

(Serving: 6, Cooking time: 40 Minutes, Difficulty: Normal)

Ingredients:

- 1/8 leek

- 100g chicken breast fillet

- 1 clove of garlic

- Curry powder, salt & cayenne pepper

- 1 tbsp olive oil

- Some lemon juice

- Some chives

- Some parmesan

- 1 avocado

- Some soy yogurt

Instructions:

1. Wash, clean, and cut the leek into rings. Rinse the chicken in cold water and cut into small pieces.

2. Peel and finely chop the garlic and mix with the chicken, curry, salt, and cayenne pepper.

3. Heat the oil in a pan. Fry the leek and chicken mixture over medium heat for 4–5 minutes. Take off the heat, let cool, and season to taste.

4. Wash the chives, shake dry and cut into rolls. Grate the parmesan.

5. Halve and core the avocado.

6. Put some of the yoghurt and the parmesan in each avocado half. Spread the chicken mixture on top and sprinkle with chives.

Kale Stilton Soup

(Serving: 6, Cooking time: 30 Minutes, Difficulty: Easy)

Ingredients:

- 1 tbsp olive oil

- 2 shallots, peeled and diced

- 2 leeks, cut and sliced

- 150 g white potatoes, peeled and diced

- 500 ml vegetable stock, fresh

- 500 ml of boiling water

- 400 g kale leaves, stems removed and roughly chopped

- 2 tbsp (30 ml) Sherry

- 200 ml skimmed milk

- 2 tbsp (30 ml) double cream (45% fat) 50 g

- Stilton, crumbled

- Large handful (20 g) parsley, roughly chopped

- Salt and freshly ground black pepper

Instructions:

1. Heat the oil in a large saucepan and gently fry the shallots and leeks for 10 minutes until tender. Stir in the potato, then add the stock and the boiling water. Bring to a boil, then reduce the heat and simmer gently for 15 minutes.

2. Use a potato masher to mash the potatoes in the pan - or mix them in a blender if you prefer. Add the kale, let it simmer gently, and cook for 4 minutes until the kale is just tender. Add the sherry, milk, cream, and half of the stilton. Let simmer until the stilton has dissolved. Season generously with salt and pepper. Divide into four bowls and serve with parsley sprinkled with Stilton.

Salsa Dip

(Serving: 4, Cooking time: 15 Minutes, Difficulty: Easy)

Ingredients:

- 1 small onion

- 1 chili pepper

- 1 clove of garlic

- 1 tbsp olive oil

- 200g chunky tomatoes

- Salt, pepper, paprika powder

- A squeeze of lemon juice

Instructions:

1. Finely dice the onion and garlic. Core the chili pepper and finely dice.

2. Heat olive oil in a pan and sauté onions, garlic and chili in it. Deglaze with canned tomatoes. Add the spices and lemon juice.

3. bring the mass to a boil. Let simmer for 5-6 minutes. Step 4. let cool and serve

Sesame chicken salad

(Serving: 2, Cooking time: 20 Minutes, Difficulty: Normal)

Ingredients:

- 1 tbsp sesame seeds

- 1 cucumber, stripped, divided lengthways, deseeded with a teaspoon and cut

- 100g infant kale, generally hacked

- 60g pakchoi, finely destroyed

- ½ red onion, finely cut

- Enormous bunch (20g) parsley, hacked

- 150g cooked chicken, destroyed

For the dressing:

- 1 tbsp additional virgin olive oil

- 1 tsp sesame oil

- Juice of 1 lime

- 1 tsp clear nectar 2 tsp soy sauce

Instructions:

1. Toast the sesame seeds in a dry frying pan for 2 minutes until delicately cooked and fragrant. Move to a plate to cool.

2. In a little bowl, combine the olive oil, sesame oil, lime juice, nectar, and soy sauce to make the dressing.

3. Place the cucumber, kale, pakchoi, red onion, and parsley in a huge bowl and tenderly combine. Pour over the dressing and blend once more.

4. Distribute the serving of salad between two plates and top with the destroyed chicken. Sprinkle over the sesame seeds not long before serving.

Kale, Tomato, Spring Onion & Pea Omelette

(Serving: 1, Cooking time: 15 Minutes, Difficulty: Normal)

Ingredients:

- 2 eggs whisked with a splash of milk

- 2 large kale leaves washed, stems removed, shredded

- 1/2 cup frozen peas

- 5 cherry tomatoes washed, halved

- 4 spring onions ends removed, washed, chopped

- 1 TBSP balsamic vinegar

Instructions:

1. As mentioned, prepare all of the ingredients.

2. In a medium-sized frying pan that has a lid, position the kale. Apply the kale to the pan with a splash of water and put the lid firmly. Cook for 2-3 mins over low-medium heat. Remove the lid after 2-3 mins, then continue to cook for a minute or until all the excess water has evaporated.

3. Slowly spill the whisked egg uniformly over the pan's base and rotate the pan to ensure equal coverage. Sprinkle the frozen peas, spring onions and dot the tomatoes over the omelette at an appropriate distance. Replace the lid and cook for around 4-5mins or until the egg is cooked through on low-medium heat.

4. As this would roast the eggs on the underside, don't be tempted to crank up the fire. Serve the omelette when still soft, as soon as the eggs are fried. When needed, season with salt & pepper and add a splash of balsamic vinegar.

Guacamole

(Serving: 5-6, Cooking time: 10 Minutes, Difficulty: Easy)

Ingredients:

- Half a ripe avocado

- 1 tomato

- 1 squirt of lemon juice

- 1 clove of garlic

- 1 half tbsp soy yogurt

- Salt and pepper

Instructions:

1. Halve the avocado and remove the stone. Remove the pulp with a spoon and mash with a fork.

2. Finely dice the tomatoes and garlic. Mix both with the lemon juice and the soy yogurt. Season to taste with salt and pepper.

Kale Muffins

(Serving: 12, Cooking time: 30 Minutes, Difficulty: Normal)

Ingredients:

- 40 g pine nuts

- 200 g flour 40 g jumbo oats

- 2 teaspoons of baking soda

- ½ teaspoon soda bicarbonate

- 1 teaspoon salt

- Freshly ground black pepper

- 60 g strong cheddar cheese, grated

- 100 g kale leaves, stems removed and finely chopped

- 2 large eggs

- 250 g yogurt

- 4 tbsp olive oil

- 100 g tomatoes, roughly chopped

- 20 g olives, pitted and roughly chopped

Instructions:

1. Preheat the oven to 200 ° C (180 ° C fan/gas 6) and line a muffin pan with 12 muffin bowls. Put the pine nuts in a dry pan and heat on high. Shake the pan gently every 30 seconds until the pine nuts are lightly toasted. Let cool down.

2. Mix the flour, oats, baking powder, soda bicarbonate, salt, pepper, cheddar, kale, and pine nuts well in a large bowl. In another bowl, whisk the eggs lightly with a fork. Add the yogurt, olive oil, tomatoes, and olives. Mix well.

3. Pour the egg mixture over the flour and fold in until it is coarsely mixed. Scoop the mixture into the muffin pan and bake for 18 to 20 minutes until a skewer set in the least browned muffin comes out clean. Let cool in the can for 5 minutes, then transfer to a cooling shelf to cool completely. Best to eat within 2 days or freeze and thaw as needed.

Cauliflower pizza with smoked salmon

(Serving: 2-4, Cooking time: 1 Hour 20 Minutes, Difficulty: Normal)

Ingredients:

• 150g cauliflower

• 125g grated cheese

• 1 egg yolk

• 1 teaspoon oregano

• 50g almond flour

• 75g ricotta

• 150g smoked salmon

• 125g prawns

• 2 tbsp pine nuts

• 1 tbsp horseradish

• Salt pepper

Instructions:

1. Preheat the oven to 180 degrees. Cut the cauliflower into florets and cook in salted water for about 10 minutes.

2. Mash the cauliflower with a potato masher. Add the grated cheese, egg yolk, chia seeds, oregano, and almond flour— season with salt and pepper. Mix everything until you get a batter.

3. Roll out the dough between two sheets of parchment paper with a rolling pin. Remove the upper arch and place the dough on a baking sheet and bake at 180 degrees for 15-20 minutes.

4. Spread the ricotta on the dough. Lay the salmon, shrimp, and pine nuts on top. Garnish with freshly grated horseradish.

Beverages & Drinks

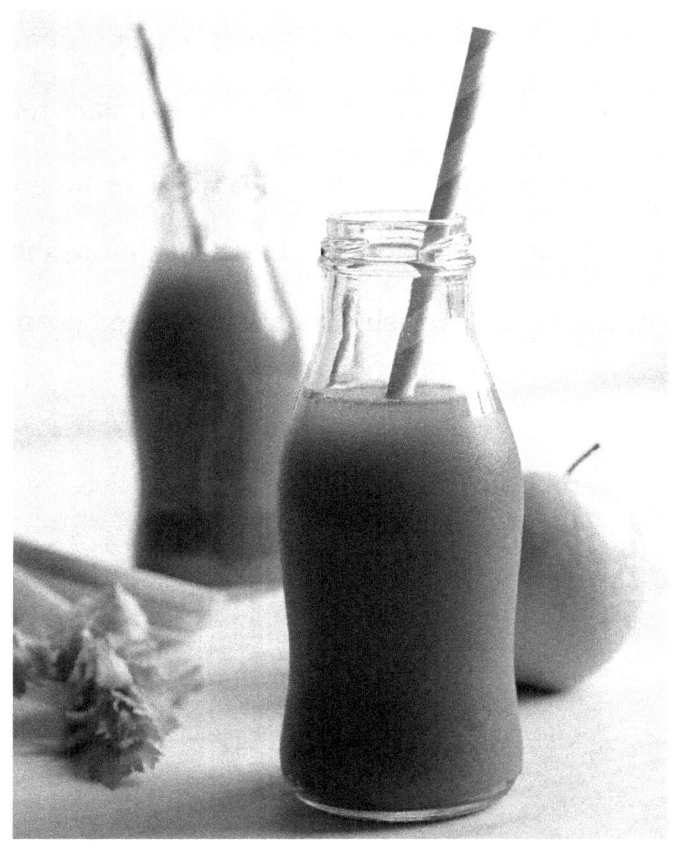

Go green smoothie

(Serving: 1 Cooking time: 15 Minutes, Difficulty: Easy)

Ingredients:

- 200 ml orange juice

- ¼ cucumber with skin

- 1 great property of kale

- 1 prize cinnamon

- 1 apple

- 1 piece of ginger

- 1 pear

Instructions:

1. Mix all ingredients smoothly and serve.

Classic Sirt juice

(Serving: 1 Cooking time: 15 Minutes, Difficulty: Easy)

Ingredients:

- 2 handfuls (75 g) kale Handful (30g) arugula

- 5 g parsley 150 g green celery (2-3 stalks)

- ½ green apple ½ lemon - juiced

- ½ teaspoon matcha powder (green tea)

Instructions:

1. Juice ingredients, should have made 250ml (1 cup) once enough for 1 juice.

2. Add matcha powder, shake or stir to combine and drink.

Juicy smoothie

(Serving: 1 Cooking time: 15 Minutes, Difficulty: Normal)

Ingredients:

* 150 ml of water or coconut water

* 1 slice of lemon with peel

* 1 banana

* 1 large key spinach

* 1 apple Juice of 1 orange

* ¼ avocado without stone

Instructions:

1. Mix all ingredients smoothly and serve.

Snacks & Desserts Recipes

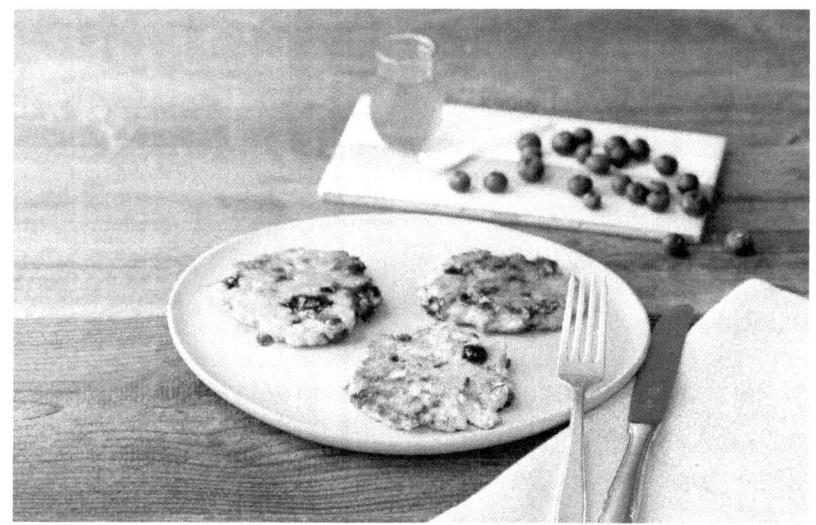

Fried chili tofu

(Serving: 1, Cooking time: 20 minutes, Difficulty: Easy)

Ingredients:

• 150 g firm tofu, cut into cubes

• 1 clove of garlic, peeled and crushed juice of

• ½ lemon

• ½ teaspoon chili flakes

• ½ teaspoon paprika

• ½ teaspoon ground turmeric

• Salt and freshly ground black pepper

• 1 teaspoon oil

Instructions:

1. Spread the tofu on a plate with kitchen paper. Cover with kitchen paper and set aside to dry. Put the garlic, lemon juice, spices, and a generous spice mixture of salt and pepper in a wide bowl.

2. Mix everything together before adding the tofu and mix gently so that the tofu is completely covered.

3. Let stand for 5 to 15 minutes. Heat the oil in a pan over medium-high heat and wait until the pan is hot before removing the tofu from the marinade and adding it to the pan. Fry for 3–4 minutes, stirring every minute, until the tofu is golden brown all over. Turn off the heat, add the remaining marinade to the pan and serve.

Lovage Ice Cream

(Servings: 1 Cook Time 20 minutes, Chilling Time 1 day,

Difficulty: Normal)

Ingredients:

• 1 cups bunch lovage, leaves and stems, roughly

chopped, about 8 stems or 2 3 wide strips of lime zest

• 2 2/3 cups whole milk

• 1 1/2 tablespoons corn-starch

• 4 tablespoons cream cheese, softened

• 1 1/2 cups heavy cream

• 3/4 cup sugar

• 1/4 cup glucose or corn syrup

• 1/4 teaspoon kosher salt

Instructions:

1. Whisk the cream cheese in a large mixing bowl until creamy. Only put aside. Mix a few teaspoons of milk with the cornstarch in a little bowl to create a little slurry. In a large saucepan over medium-high heat, mix the remaining milk, cream, sugar, glucose or corn syrup, and salt. Please bring it to a boil and cook for 5 minutes or so. Remove from the fire and whisk in a slurry of cornstarch.

2. Apply the passion and the zest of lime. Return to the stove over medium-high heat and return to boiling heat, stirring continuously for around 1 minute, until gently thickened. Remove from the heat and pour the cream cheese over the mixture and whisk until thoroughly mixed.

3. Cover and refrigerate overnight, until thoroughly chilled, letting the lovage begin to steep. In an ice cream maker, go through a fine-mesh strainer and process. Pack it into a storage bowl and freeze until concrete for several hours.

No-Bake Triple Berry Mini Tarts

(Serving: 6, Cooking time: 20 minutes, Difficulty: Easy)

Ingredients:

- Frozen mixed berries, defrosted – 1 cup

- Honey - .5 cup

- Cacao butter, melted – 5 tablespoons

- Coconut cream - .33 cup

- Walnuts, raw – 2 cups

- Dates – 1 cup

Instructions:

1. In a food processor combine the walnuts with the dates until it forms a crumbly mixture that can hold together when you press it. Scrape down the sides as needed.

2. Prepare a mini muffin tin for the crust, to make the mini tarts. Spray the pan with non-stick cooking spray.

3. Press the prepared crust into the mini muffin tin, forming mini tarts with crust pressed both on the bottom and on the sides of the muffin cups.

4. In a blender, mix the berries and other remaining ingredients until completely smooth. Divide the berry mixture between the crusts.

5. Place the filled muffin tin in the fridge and allow it to chill for six hours, or until set.

6. Use a kitchen knife to run around the edges of each tart to release them from the pan. Use a fork and take each tart out of the pan. Serve or store in a container in the fridge or freezer.

Cherry Cream

(Servings: 4 Cook time: 2 hours, Difficulty: Normal)

Ingredients:

- 2 c. cherries, pitted and chopped

- 1 c. almond milk

- ½ c. whipping cream

- 3 eggs, whisked

- 1/3 c. stevia

- 1 tsp. lemon juice

- ½ tsp. vanilla extract

Instructions:

1. In your food processor, combine the cherries with the milk and the rest of the ingredients, pulse well, divide into cups and keep in the fridge for 2 hours before serving.

Buckwheat Chocolate Pudding

(Servings: 2 Cook Time 15 Minutes, Difficulty: Normal)

Ingredients:

- Buckwheat pudding

- 70 g buckwheat previously soaked in water for a couple of hours

- 200 ml rice milk 50 g dates previously soaked in water for

- 1 hour 50 g coconut cream the thickened cream from a can of full-fat coconut milk

- 100 g banana ripe

- 20 g raw cacao powder

- 130 ml rice milk

- 1 tablespoon agave for extra sweetness

Toppings:

- Coconut whipped cream blueberries

Instructions:

1. Rinse it well until the buckwheat has been soaked, then let it drip thoroughly. Please put it in a small saucepan with 200 ml of almond milk or a medium saucepan.

2.   Just get it to a boil. Drop the heat to a low stage, cover and cook for approx. Fifteen mins.

2. Withdraw from the sun. Drain it if there is any liquid left and let it cool off entirely. Drain the dates and drop them in the mixer. All the other ingredients are added: cooked buckwheat, coconut milk, banana, cacao powder, approx. 130 ml of milk with rice. Blend until smooth and creamy. Add a little more almond milk if the mixture is too thick before achieving the perfect consistency.

3. If needed, change the sweetness by adding 1-tablespoon of agave syrup. Serve with coconut whipped cream and blueberries in jars and cover it.

Honey-Roasted Plums with Ricotta

(Serving: 4, Cooking time: 20 minutes, Difficulty: Easy)

Ingredients:

- Plums, halved and pitted – 4

- Butter, melted – 1 tablespoon

- Honey – .25 cup

- Ricotta, part-skim, ideally fresh – 1 cup

Instructions:

1. Begin by setting your oven to Fahrenheit four-hundred degrees and preparing a baking dish or skillet that can fit all eight plum halves. Add the melted butter into the dish.

2. Arrange your plum halves in the prepared dish, with the cut side facing upward. Drizzle the honey over the plums and bake until the plums are soft and release the juices, about fifteen minutes.

3. If you want to slightly char the plums, you can turn the broiler on for the last minute of baking.

4. Divide the roasted plums between serving dishes and top them with the ricotta. Serve while still warm.

Sirt date pudding with toffee sauce

(Serving: 2-6 Cooking Time: 30 Minutes, Difficulty: Normal)

Ingredients:

*   250 g pitted Medjool dates

*   2 tsp bicarbonate soda

*   200 g of ground walnuts

*   50 g buckwheat flour, sifted

*   100 g unsalted butter or coconut oil plus a little more

for greasing

For the toffee sauce:

*   200 ml coconut cream

*   100 g pitted Medjool dates 150 ml water

*   75 g unsalted butter or coconut oil

Instructions:

1. Preheat the oven to 1700C / 31⁄2 coal. Grease lightly with a 20 cm square baking pan. Pour 200 ml of boiling water over the pudding dates and let them soak for 5–10 minutes. Place the dates and their soaking liquid in a food processor after soaking, and blend 7-8 times or until you have a coarse paste.

2. Apply the baking soda and blend again. Apply the walnuts, flour, and butter to the surface. Flash until there's a sweet, smooth paste for you. In the prepared pan, scoop the mixture, flatten the lid, and then throw it into the oven and bake for 30 minutes. (It can come out clean if you poke the middle with a wooden skewer.) When the cake is baking, make the sauce.

3. In a small saucepan, place all the ingredients and bring them to a boil. Remove from the heat and set aside to cool a little for 5-10 minutes, then add a smooth sauce. You can need to apply some water if it is too thick, depending on the type of coconut cream you are using. Return the sauce to the saucepan and serve over the warm pudding until the pudding is ready.

Olive tapenade

(Serving: 4, Cooking time: 20 minutes, Difficulty: Easy)

Ingredients:

- 1 clove of garlic, peeled and crushed peel

- Juice of ½ lemon

- 1 tbsp capers

- Drain 3 anchovy fillets, chop them up

- Drain 200 g pitted green or black olives and roughly chop

- 2 tbsp extra virgin olive oil

Instructions:

1. Put the garlic, lemon peel and juice, capers and anchovies in a food processor and stir until smooth.

2. Add the olives and mix again. Do not overmix as some pieces of olive will ensure a good consistency. Scoop out the paste and stir in the olive oil. The tapenade stays in the refrigerator for a few days.

CPSIA information can be obtained
at www.ICGtesting.com
Printed in the USA
BVHW051557130421
604814BV00004B/854